Meriam Khadhar
Manel Aoun
Fares Azaiz

Nephropathy associated with contrast media

Meriam Khadhar
Manel Aoun
Fares Azaiz

Nephropathy associated with contrast media

and if we injected ourselves with kidney poison

ScienciaScripts

Imprint

Any brand names and product names mentioned in this book are subject to trademark, brand or patent protection and are trademarks or registered trademarks of their respective holders. The use of brand names, product names, common names, trade names, product descriptions etc. even without a particular marking in this work is in no way to be construed to mean that such names may be regarded as unrestricted in respect of trademark and brand protection legislation and could thus be used by anyone.

Cover image: www.ingimage.com

This book is a translation from the original published under ISBN 978-620-6-72364-6.

Publisher:
Sciencia Scripts
is a trademark of
Dodo Books Indian Ocean Ltd. and OmniScriptum S.R.L publishing group

120 High Road, East Finchley, London, N2 9ED, United Kingdom
Str. Armeneasca 28/1, office 1, Chisinau MD-2012, Republic of Moldova, Europe
Printed at: see last page
ISBN: 978-620-8-24570-2

Contents

Chapter 1

Acute renal failure (ARF) associated with iodinated contrast media (ICPs) is a feared complication that occurs after many radiological procedures. These explorations regularly expose an increasing number of patients to the nephrotoxic potential of ICPs [1].

Iodine contrast media-associated nephropathy (ICPN) is an acute renal failure that typically occurs between 24 and 72 hours after an injection of ICP [1].

While the vast majority of cases of acute renal impairment often develop after standard radiological examinations, this complication is increasingly encountered in interventional cardiology, and specifically in the management of coronary artery disease, where vascular opacification with PCI is the only diagnostic and therapeutic alternative in most cases [2].

AKI associated with PCI is the third most common cause of acute in-hospital renal failure after functional AKI and drug-induced causes [3]. Among the reasons cited are the increased use of cardiac catheterisation techniques, multiple comorbidities in patients undergoing percutaneous coronary intervention and the use of larger quantities of PCI for complex coronary lesions.

The incidence of this complication varies considerably depending on pre-existing risk factors and the characteristics of the examination.

The incidence is estimated to be 1 to 2% in the general population, rising progressively with risk factor(s), reaching almost 50% in patients with multiple risk factors [4], notably diabetes and chronic renal failure following coronary angiography or percutaneous coronary intervention [2].

Its occurrence in the cardiology setting is associated with increased hospitalisation time and costs, as well as increased cardiovascular morbidity and mortality [5].

Prevention is therefore one of the main therapeutic challenges.

Three international recommendations concerning the diagnosis, prevention and management of CINP have been published: those of the European Society of Urogenital Radiology (ESUR)[6], those of the Kidney Disease: Improvement of Global Outcome (KDIGO) initiative[7], and finally those of the European Renal Best Practice (ERBP)[8]. It should be pointed out that these recommendations are the result of the interpretation of studies of varying quality on diverse populations, most of which are ambulatory. Consequently, the practitioner should apply them with caution, taking into account the particular clinical context of each patient[4].

Acute renal failure has been largely under-reported in North Africa, with a few studies reported in Tunisia where the incidence of ARF associated with contrast media varies from 8.8% to 17.2% [9] [10] depending on the study.

This prompted us to carry out a study with the following objectives:

❖Determining the incidence of ARF associated with contrast products

❖Identifying predictive factors for the occurrence of ARF associated with iodinated contrast media in the cardiology setting.

Chapter 2

1. Type of study :

This is a retrospective descriptive and analytical observational study of 133 patients who underwent coronary angiography and/or coronary angioplasty in the cardiology department of the Mongi Slim Hospital over a 3-month period from April to June 2023.

2. Methods

1.1 Inclusion criteria

The patients included in this study were :

Ages over 18

Having undergone coronary angiography and/or coronary angioplasty at the cardiology department of the Mongi Slim Hospital during the study period

1.2 Non-inclusion criteria :

The criteria for non-inclusion were:

Patients with obstructive renal failure

Chronic dialysis patients

1.3 Exclusion criteria

Patients with missing data in the file were excluded:

In whom we do not have pre- and post-procedural creatinine (48h- 72h after the procedure)

Whose estimated left ventricular ejection fraction (LVEF) was not mentioned

2 Data collection

An information sheet has been drawn up in advance (Appendix) to specify the following data:

2.1 Epidemiological data

Age

Sex

2.2 Anamnestic data

Habits: smoking.

Medical   history (cardiovascular risk factors): diabetes, hypertension, pre-existing nephropathy, dyslipidemia, etc.

 History of heart failure

 Previous injections of iodine contrast product (ICP)

 Medications: Metformin, aminoglycosides, diuretics, renin angiotensin system blockers (RASBs), non-steroidal anti-inflammatory drugs (NSAIDs), statins, proton pump inhibitors (PPIs) and gliflozins (or sodium-glucose co-transporter type 2 (SGLT2) inhibitors).

2.3 Clinical data

 Systolic blood pressure (SBP) and diastolic blood pressure (DBP)

 s state of hydration.

2.4 Biological data

 The day before the procedure: blood creatinine, urea, ionogram, CBC.

 Between the $2^{\text{ère}}$ and the $3^{\text{ère}}$ day after the procedure: blood creatinine.

2.5 Echo-cardiographic data

Left ventricular ejection fraction (LVEF).

The state of the inferior vena cava

2.6 Procedural data

2.6.1 Vindication of the procedure

> Persistent ST-segment elevation myocardial infarction (STEMI)

> Coronary syndrome (ACS) ST(-) Troponin (+)

> Angorstable

> SCAST(-)Troponin(-)

> Preoperative coronary angiography,

> Assessment of dilated cardiomyopathy (DCM),

> Assessment of a double rhythm (TR)

> Elective angioplasty

> Assessment of acute heart failure

> Myocardial scintigraphy or stress test or positive coronal CT scan *2.6.2 Nature of the procedure*

> Coronary angiography,

> Coronary angioplasty

> Coronary angiography and ad-hoc coronary angioplasty

> Coronary angiography and primary angioplasty

2.6.3 The time between [hospital admission and [angiocoronary angiography

- Emergency coronary angiography (< 24 hours)

- Scheduled coronary angiography

2.6.4 Clinical data at the time of Гexamen

Blood pressure at the time of the operation: per procedural hypotension and possible use of vasoactive amines

2.6.5 Data relating to iodine contrast media

Nature and quantity of the contrast medium to be injected

2.7 Results of coronary angiography :

Monotruncal, bi-truncal and tri-truncal coronary disease

Normal or infiltrated coronary network

2.8 Mehran's score

We calculated the Mehran score for all patients.

2.9 Prevention protocol

2.9.1 Nature and volume of contrast agent administered

Intravascular contrast products are based on a tri-iodine heterocyclic benzene ring which gives them their radiopacity (figure 1).

The overall structure can be a monomer (1 single benzene ring) or a dimer (2 benzene rings). A distinction is made between ionic and non-ionic molecules according to their association with a sodium or meglumine cation.

ICPs are also classified according to their osmolality and viscosity[ll].

In our study, two ICPs were used:

J Iohexol (Omnipaque 350) was available at the hospital.

It is a non-ionic monomer with a low osmolarity (780 mOsm/kg H20 at 37°C) corresponding to 350 mg of iodine element per millilitre and a viscosity of 10.6

m Pasa37°C[12].

J Iodinaxol (Visipaque 320) was reserved, when available, mainly for stage 3, 4 or 5 renal failure patients.

It is an iso osmolar non-ionic dimer. (290 mOsm/kg H2O at 37°C) corresponding to 320 mg of iodine element per millilitre and having a viscosity of 11.4 m Pasa37°C[13].

Unfortunately, iodinaxol was not always available at the hospital.

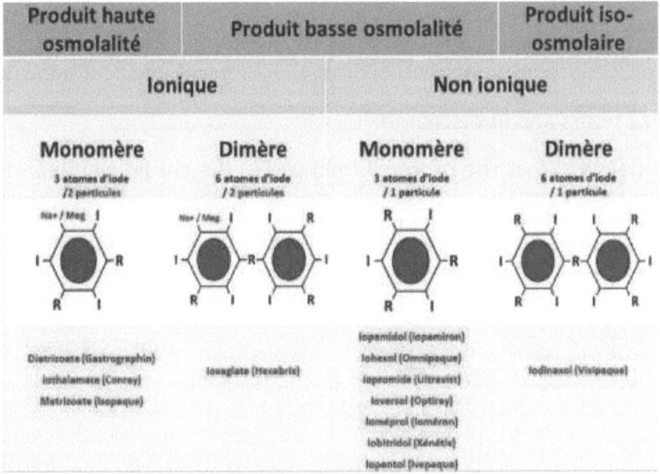

Figure 1: Structure of iodine contrast products

We calculated two predictive ratios for the occurrence of ARF associated with PCI :

❖ The ratio of injected volume to creatinine clearance.

❖ The ratio of iodine dose in grams to creatinine clearance.

2.9.2 Protocol adopted in the cardiology department and patient follow-up

No preventive measures were recommended for patients explored in emergency.

Prevention protocols were applied to at-risk patients: specifically diabetics and/or patients suffering from renal failure.

In patients who presented for an elective or scheduled procedure with a satisfactory state of hydration, strategic prevention was started 24 hours before injection of the iodine contrast medium, based on intravenous administration of one litre of 9g/L NaCL while respecting the hemodynamic state of patients with left ventricular (LV) dysfunction in order to avoid pulmonary overload. We did not use bicarbonate-based solutions.

Rehydration was continued on the day of the procedure and for 48 hours afterwards, with strict monitoring of hemodynamic status and signs of overload.

After the procedure, patients had clinical checks and biological measurements within 48-72 hours and at discharge.

The figure below shows the protocol followed in the cardiology department of the Mongi Slim Hospital.

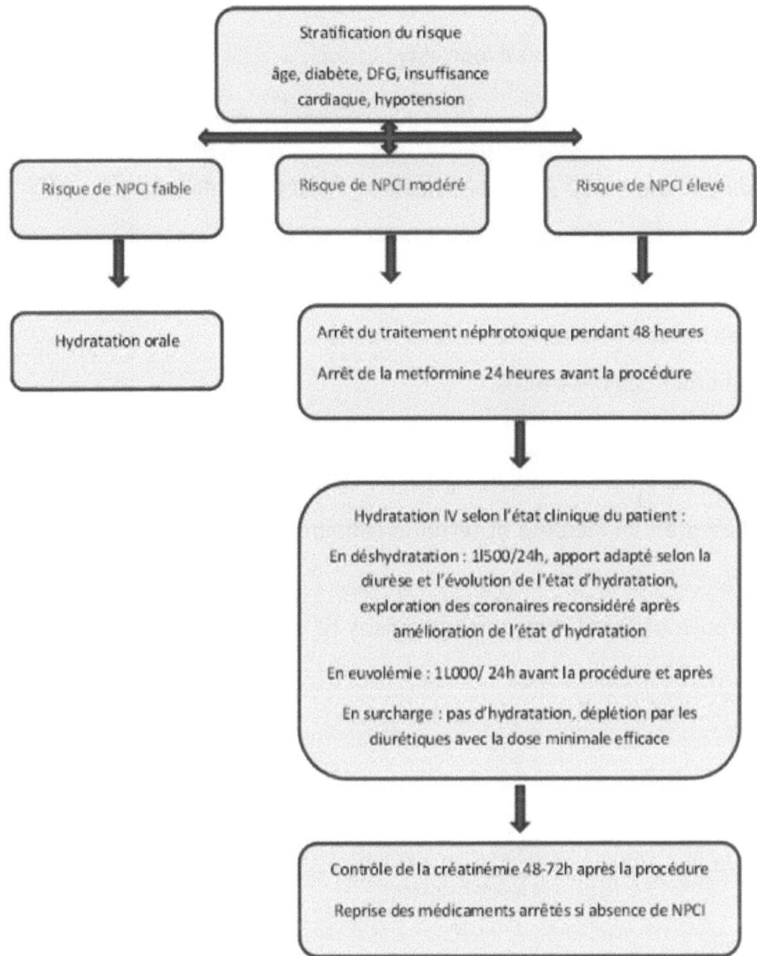

Figure 2: The strategic preventive approach adopted by the cardiology department at Mongi Slim Hospital

2.10 Evolving data

The assessment criterion was the occurrence of NPCI by analysing its factors associated risks.

In cases of ARF associated with ICPs, we have noted :

The degree of severity of IRA according to the KDIGOs

Clinical consequences: OAP - diuresis breakdown - hydrolytic disorders

The use of extra renal epuration

The subsequent evolution of renal function: total/partial recovery/no recovery

Length of stay and in-hospital mortality

2.11 Definitions

<u>*Contrast-induced nephropathy (CIN):</u>

According to the KDIGO 2012 classification [7], NPCI is defined as:

An increase of **more than 44 umol/l (>=** 0.5 mg/dl) in creatinemia,

and/or a relative increase of **more than 25%** of the base value,

within 48 hours of PCI injection

without other obvious causes.

<u>*IRA KDIGO ;</u>

The classification of ARF according to the KDIGO 2012 international guidelines [7] is based on an increase in serum creatinine and/or a decrease in diuresis (Table I).

The purpose of these recommendations is to characterise the severity of an ARI.

<u>Table I: Classification of acute renal failure according to the KDIGO international recommendations</u>

Stadium	Plasma creatinine	Diurese
1	> 26.5 pmol/l or 1.5 to 1.9 times baseline plasma creatinine	< 0.5 ml/kg/h for 6 to 12 hours.
2	2.0 to 2.9 times baseline plasma creatinine	< 0.5 ml/kg/h for > 12h
3	3.0 times baseline plasma creatinine or plasma creatinine > 354 pmol/l or initiation of extra-renal purification	< 0.3 ml/kg/h for > 24h or anuria for > 12h

<u>*Glomerular filtration rate :</u>

Glomerular filtration rate (GFR) was estimated using the MDRD (Modification ofdiet in renal disease) formula (Figure 2)[14].

$$\text{eDFG} = 1\,75 \times (S_{cr} \times 0.01\,13)^{\cdot 154} \times \text{age}^{-.0203} \times 0.742$$
$$\text{(if female)} \times 1.21\,2 \text{ (if black)}$$

<u>Figure 3: MDRD formula for calculating glomerular filtration rate</u>

<u>***Chronic renal failure :**</u>

Chronic renal failure (CRF) has been defined as a GFR of less than 60ml/min/1.73m^2 body surface area for at least 3 months [7].

The stages of chronic kidney disease have been defined by the KDIGO 2012 working group [7] (Table I).

Table II: Stages of chronic kidney disease

Stadium	GFR (ml/min/1.73 m^2 SC)	Definition
1	>90	Chronic kidney disease* with normal or increased GFR**.
2	60-89	Chronic kidney disease* with slightly reduced GFR
3	30-59	Chronic moderate renal failure
4	15-29	Severe chronic renal failure
5	<15	Chronic end-stage renal failure

* With markers of renal impairment: clinical prot^inuria, k^maturia, leucocyturia, or morphological or histological abnormalities, or markers of tubular dysfunction, persisting for more than three months *DFG: Glomerular filtration rate

<u>***The Mehran clinical score for predicting the risk of nephropathy associated with iodine contrast products:**</u>

The NPCI risk score used in our study was that validated by Mehran et al [15] (Table II).

Table III: Mehran score for predicting the risk of nephropathy associated with iodine contrast products

Variables	Points
Arterial hypotension	5
Use of a counter-pulse ball	5
Congestive heart failure	5
Age > 75	4
serum creatinine > 133 umol/l or eGFR < 60ml/min/1.73 m^2	4
eGFR [40-60[	2
eGFR [20-40[	4
eGFR<20	6
Diabetes	3

Anemie	3
Volume of iodine contrast medium administered *	1

*1 point for each lOOcc of PCI administered

The risk is considered:

- Lowilescore<5.
- Moderate if the score is between 6 and 10.
- High if the score is between 11 and 15.
- Treselevesilescore>16.

***Arterial hypotension** is defined as a SAP <80 mmHg for > 1 hour, requiring the use of inotropes or placement of a counterpulsation balloon within 24 hours [15].

***Congestive heart failure** has been defined as heart failure symptomatic of dyspnea classed as Ш/W according to the New York Heart Association classification and/or antecedents of pulmonary redeme [15].

***Diabetes** was defined as fasting blood glucose >126 mg/dL, random blood glucose >200 mg/dL, glycated haemoglobin >6.5% or if there had been a previous diagnosis or specific anti-diabetic treatment administered since admission [16].

***Anemia** has been defined exclusively on the basis of hemoglobin measurement according to the World Health Organisation (WHO)[17].

***** <13g/dl in men,

***** <12g/dl in women.

***Arterial hypertension :**

Arterial hypertension (AH) has been defined, according to WHO, as a SBP > 140 mmHg and/or DBP > 90 mmHg confirmed on several occasions or the use of antihypertensive treatment [18].

*** <u>Left ventricular dysfunction :</u>**

Left ventricular dysfunction is defined as LVEF < 50%.

Moderately reduced LVEF is defined as a value between 40% and 49% and reduced LVEF as a value below 40% [19].

*** <u>Dehydration:</u>**

Dehydration corresponds to a reduction in the volume of water in the extra and/or intra cellular sector.

J <u>Extracellular dehydration</u> [20]:

<u>Clinical:</u> weight loss, skin folds, hypotonia of the eyeballs, orthostatic arterial hypotension, oliguria, tachycardia.

<u>Biology:</u> indirect biological signs reflecting a decrease in extracellular volume: hemoconcentration syndrome: elevated protidemia, elevated hematocrit, collapsed natriuresis, elevated creatinemia, elevated plasma urea, hyperuricemia, "contraction" metabolic alkalosis.

J <u>Intra-cellular dehydration</u> [21]:

<u>Clinical:</u> thirst, dry mucous membranes, weight loss, neuropsychological signs (agitation, confusion, convulsion, coma, etc.)

<u>Biology:</u> hypernatremia, hyperosomolalite

***<u>State of overload/hyper-volmia ;</u>**

Peripheral redemas, signs of pulmonary congestion, arterial hypertension or jugular stasis (turgidity, hepato-jugular reflux) may be markers of hyperthrombosis [22].

3. Statistical analysis of data

Data entry and statistical analysis were carried out using SPSS version 23 software.

The nature of the distribution of each quantitative variable was checked using the Kolmogorov-Smirnov (K-S) test.

3.1. Descriptive study

For the qualitative variables, we calculated the simple frequencies (n) and the relative frequencies (as a percentage).

For quantitative variables, we calculated the means (M) or the medians (Med), the standard deviations (SD) and/or the range (Extreme values: Minimum (Min) and Maximum (Max)).

3.2. Analytical study

The search for factors associated with the occurrence of ARF associated with ICPs was carried out in analysis :

-Univariee: par etude de (association entre :

* two qualitative variables using Pearson's Chi-square test and Fisher's exact test. In the case of a significant association, the risk of the occurrence of this NPCI was calculated using the Odds ratio (OR).

*a qualitative variable and a quantitative variable using:

For quantitative variables with a normal distribution, Student's t-test.

Non-parametric tests were used for variables with a non-Gaussian distribution. ROC curves were constructed for quantitative variables that were significantly associated with a NPCI. We chose as the threshold the value offering the best compromise between sensitivity and specificity. This is the threshold at which the ROC curve shows a point of inflection.

-Multivariate: using the cox regression model. The significance level was set at 0.05 or 5%.

4. Bibliographic research

The bibliographic search was carried out using the Pubmed, Google Scholar and Science Direct websites and search engines.

We studied literature in English and French.

The keywords used were: acute renal failure, iodine contrast medium, coronary angiography, angioplasty, prevention, risk factor.

Bibliographic references were managed using Zotero software.

5. Ethical considerations

In our study, we declare that there is no conflict of interest.

Data relating to the identity of patients has been carefully processed in order to respect their anonymity.

Chapter 3

1 DESCRIPTIVE STUDY

1.1 Sample size

Our study population consisted of 133 patients.

1.2 Epidemiological data on the study population

1.2.1 Age

The median age of the patients studied was 63, with extremes ranging from 28 to 82 .

The age group between 50 and 69 was the most represented, accounting for 69% of the population studied (Figure 4).

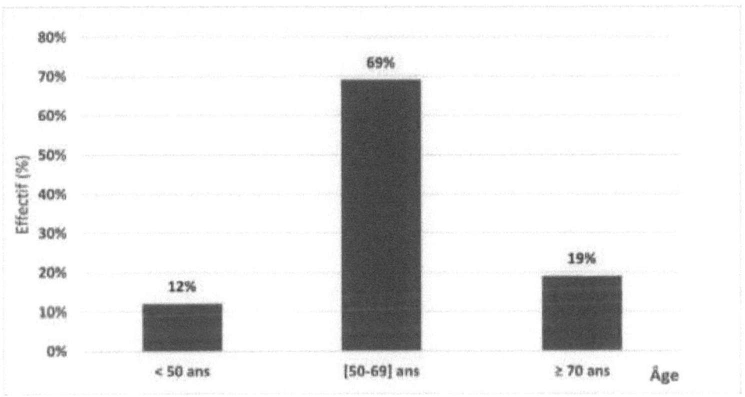

Figure 4: Breakdown of the study population by age group

1.2.2 Gender

The population studied comprised 93 men (70%) and 40 women (30%), giving a sex ratio of 2.33 (Figure 4).

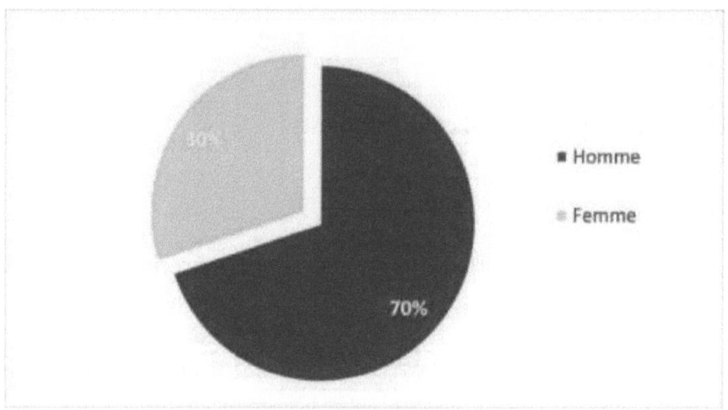

1.3 Anamnestic data on the study population

1.3.1 Habits

Seventy patients were active smokers (53%)

1.3.2 Medical history

1.3.2.1 Diabetes

Diabetes was noted in 67 patients (50% of the population). Among these diabetic patients, 38 patients had insulin-requiring diabetes (57%).

of the diabetic population) (Figure 6).

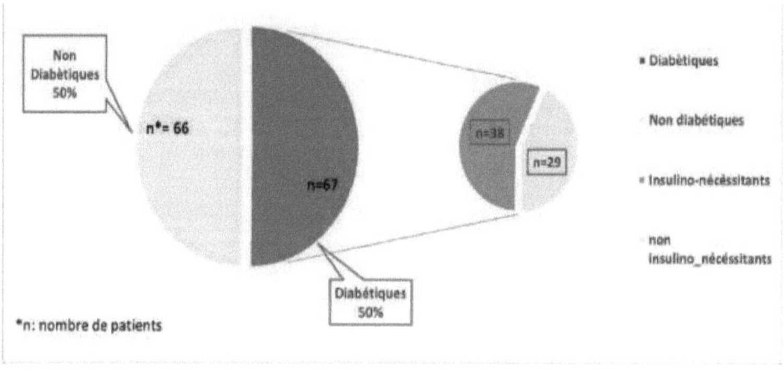

1.3.2.2 Arterial hypertension

High blood pressure was noted in 78 patients (59%).

Table IV below shows the distribution of hypertensive patients according to the antihypertensive treatment used.

Table V: Anti-hypertensive treatments in hypertensive patients

Treatment	Number n (% of hypertensives)
No	13 (17%)
BSRA* + diuretics	26 (33%)
BSRA* alone	31 (40%)
Diuretics alone	8 (10%)
ARB: Angiotensin-Renin System Blockers	

1.3.2.3   Dyslipidemia

Dyslipidemia was present in 45 patients (34% of the population).

1.3.2.4   Pre-existing kidney disease

In our study, nine patients (7% of the sample) were being monitored for chronic kidney disease. All were associated with diabetic nephropathy.

Eight of these patients had CKD: six had a creatinine clearance of between 30 and 59 ml/min/l,73m^2 and two patients had severe chronic renal failure with a creatinine clearance of less than 30 ml/min/l,73m .^{2}

1.3.2.5 Number of cardiovascular risk factors

In our study, we found that 114 patients had two or more cardiovascular risk factors, representing 86% of the population studied.

Table VI: Distribution of cardiovascular risk factors in the study population

Cardiovascular risk factors	Number n (% of total)
Active smoking (current or stopped less than three years ago)	70 (53%)
Age	103 (77,4%)
Men > 50	76 (81.7% of men)
Women > 60	27 (67.5% of women)
Diabetes	67 (50%)
Hypertension	78 (59%)
Dyslipidemia	45 (34%)

1.3.3 Injection of iodine contrast less than 3 months old

Twenty patients (15% of the study population) had investigations requiring the use of PCI injections (Table VII).

The median time from ICP injection to current examination was 21 days, with extremes between 3 and 109 days. Only one patient had a history of ICP injection less than 5 days old.

Type of injection		Number n (% of total)
Coronary angiography	Intra-arterial	19 (14%)
Coro scanner	Intravenous	1(1%)
Angioscan	Intravenous	0

1.3.4 History of acute renal failure

Among the population studied, 6 patients (4% of the sample) had a history of ARF, 3 of whom developed ARF following an injection of PCI (representing 15% of patients who received an injection). The etiology of ARF in the other patients is unknown.

devolution was marked by a return to baseline creatinine levels in all patients.

1.3.5 Medication concomitant with [injection of iodine contrast agent

Concomitant medication with PCI injection was taken by the entire study population.

The various treatments are listed in table IX below.

It should be noted that none of the patients in our study were taking aminoglycosides.

Medication	Workforce	Percentage
BSRA*	88	66%
Beta-agonists	101	76%
Insulin	38	29%
Metformin	21	16%
iSGLT2*	21	16%
Diuretics	66	50%

Spironolactone	17	13%
Loop diuretics	27	20%
Thiazide diuretics	22	17%
Statins	123	93%
PPI	109	82%
NSAIDS*	8	6%
Aspirin	117	88%
Clopidogrel	117	88%

*NSAIDs: non 51ëro'|д1еп5 inflammatory drugs, RASB: renin angiotensin system blockers, PPIs: proton pump inhibitors, ISGLT2: sodium-glucose co-transporter type 2 inhibitors.

1.4 Clinical data

Table IX below illustrates the pre-procedural clinical data.

Table XI: Clinical data for the study population

Number n (%)	
Signs of dehydration	6 (5%)
Signs of overload	27 (20%)
Median in mmHg (min-max)	
Systolic blood pressure	130 (70-187)
Diastolic blood pressure	75 (5-104)

1.5 Biological data

Table XII summarises the various biological data.

Table XIII: Biological data for the study population

	Mediane	IQR [25%-75%]
Hematocrit (%)	41	[37-44]
Lymphocyte (/mm)^3	1780	[1275 -2365]
Neutrophils (/mm)^3	5170	[3665-7100]
Neutrophil/lymphocyte ratio	2,9	[l,8-4,3]
Uree (mmol/l)	6,3	[4,9-7,8]
Pre-procedural creatinine (umol/l)	81	[68,6- 92,7]
Kalemia (mmol/l)	4,4	[4-4,75]
Natremia (mmol/l)	138	[136-139]
	Average +/ecarttype	Min - Max
Hemoglobin (g/dl)	13,2 +/- 2	6,6-17,5

Anemia was noted in 42 patients, i.e. 32% of the population studied.

Figure 7 below illustrates the distribution of our population according to GFR calculated from pre-procedural creatinine, showing that 27 patients (20%) had impaired renal function (GFR < 60 ml/min/l,73m^2 SC).

We do not know the etiology of renal failure.

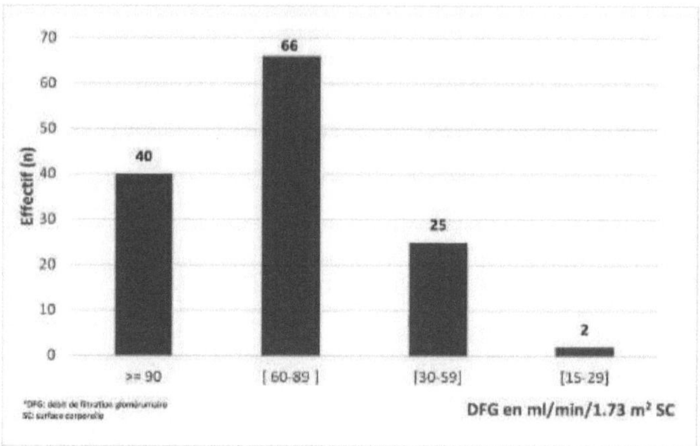

Figure 7: Population distribution by creatinine pзё procedural

1.6 Ultrasound data

The median LVEF was 55% with an IQR of 25-75 [45%-60%].

Forty-five patients (34%) had left ventricular dysfunction (Figure 7).

The inferior vena cava was dilated in 13 patients.

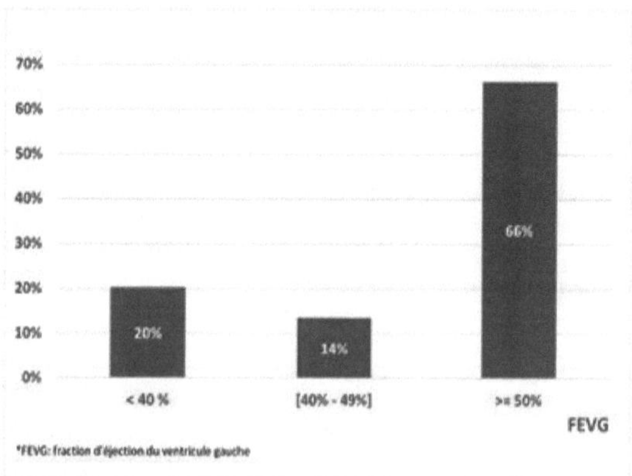

Figure 8: Distribution of the study population according to left ventricular ejection fraction

1.7 Background information

1.7.1 Indication for coronary angiography

The indications for coronary angiography were dominated by STEMI, as shown in figure 9 below.

Emergency procedures (< 24 hours) for diagnostic or therapeutic purposes accounted for 68% of investigations.

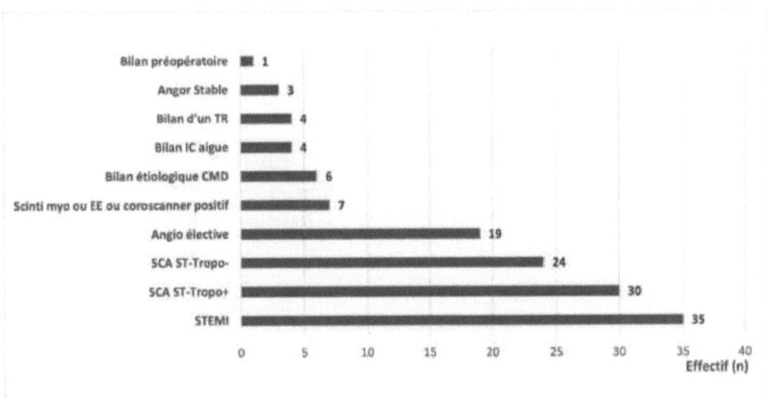

Figure 9: Distribution of the study population according to indications for coronary angiography.

1.7.2 Nature and approach of l'examen realise

Figure 10 below illustrates the nature of the examination carried out.

Fifty-four patients (41% of the population) had undergone diagnostic or non-interventional coronary angiography (without angioplasty).

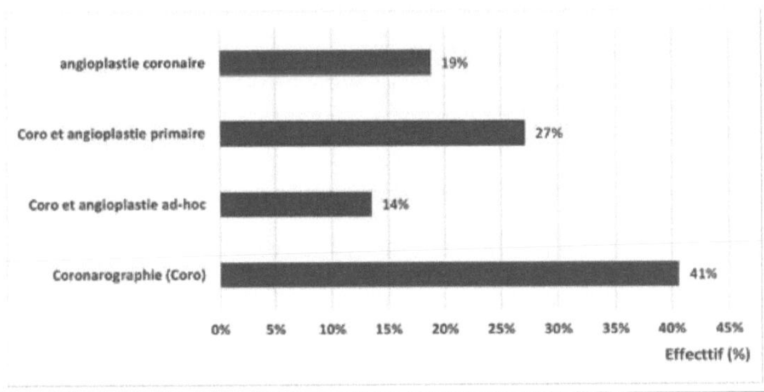

Figure 10: Breakdown of the study population by type of examination

This angiocoronary angiography was mainly performed radially (95% of cases), as shown in figure 11.

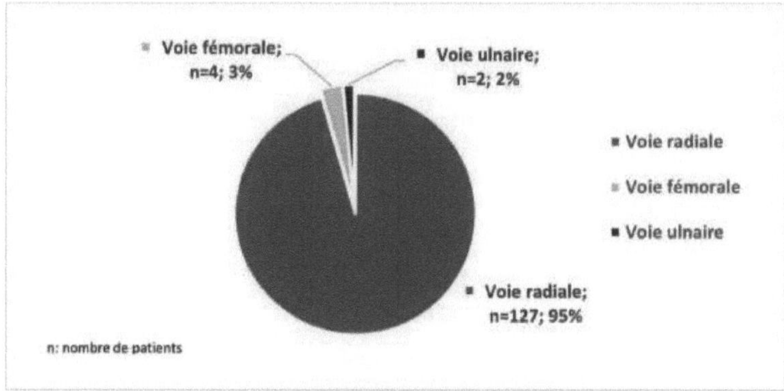

Figure 11: Distribution of the study population according to the approach used

1.7.3 From hospital admission to angio-coronary angiography

The median time between admission and angiography was 2 days, with an IQR of 25-75% [1-5 days] and extremes ranging from the day of admission (i.e. JI) to 16 days.

This delay varied according to the indications for angiography and coronary angiography.

Table XIV: Delay between hospital admission and radiological examination in the cardiology department

Time between admission and exploration

	Mediane enjours	Extreme days
STEMI and NSTEMI	2	1-11
Other indication	5	1-16

1.7.4 Clinical data at the time of the procedure

Five patients experienced per-procedural hypotension, 4 of whom required vasopressor amines following hemodynamic instability.

Digestive haemorrhage was the cause of per-procedural hypotension in only one case. No deaths occurred during the procedure.

1.7.5 PDC data

1.7.5.1 Nature of the product used

Iohexol (Omnipaque 350) was used in 126 patients (95%), while Iodinaxol (Visipaque 320) was recommended in 7 patients (5%), 4 of whom had a clearance of less than 45ml/min/l,73m2 and 3 of whom were diabetics at the CKD stage.

1.7.5.2 Quantity of product used

The median volume of PCI administered during the angiographic procedure was 100 ml, with extremes ranging from 30 to 500 ml (figure 11).

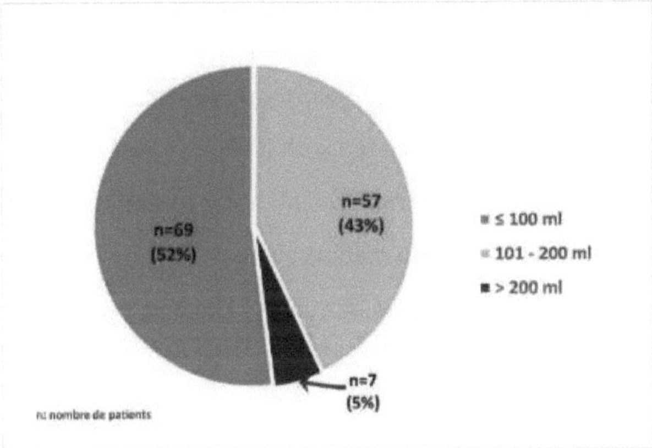

Figure 12: Distribution of the study population according to the volume of contrast medium administered

The median volume/clearance ratio was 1.3, with extremes ranging from 0.4 to 15.6 and an IQR of 25%-75% [0.7-2].

The median dose of iodine administered was 30 grams per procedure with an IQ.R of 25%-75% [18-45].

The median iodine dose ratio in grams/clearance was 0.4 with an IQR of 25%-75% [0.2-0.6].

1.8 Results of coronary angiography

We observed that bi-truncular coronary involvement was the most frequent during coronary angiography, detected in 43 patients (32%) (Figure13).

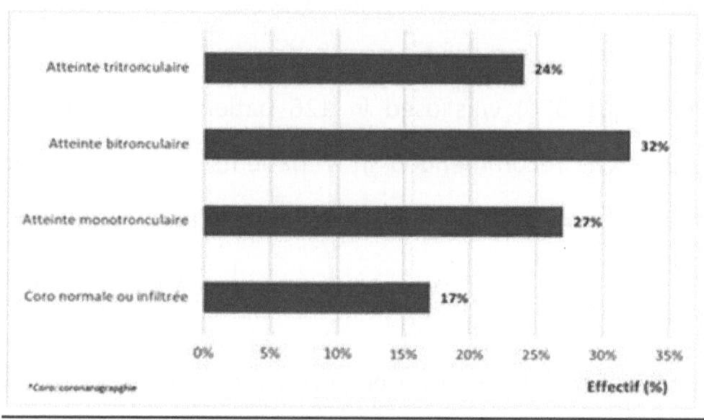

Figure 13: Coronary angiography results

1.9 Mehran score

According to the Mehran Score, the majority of patients (n=93), or 70%, were at low risk of developing AKI associated with ICPs.

Figure 14 below shows the distribution of the population according to this score, ranging from 0 to 21, with a median score of 4.

It should be noted that 9 patients in our study (7%) had a score above 11 (high and very high risk).

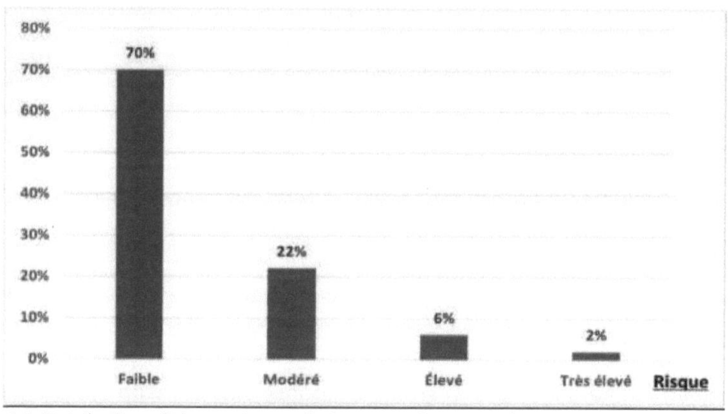

Figure 14: Distribution of the study population according to Mehran score

1.10 Evolving data

In our study population, 21 patients developed AKI associated with ICPs (16%).

1.10.1Classification of acute renal failure

According to the 2012 KDIGO classification, it was observed that among patients who developed AKI associated with PCI, 15 patients (71% of the sample) presented with stage 1 acute renal failureë, five patients (24% of the sample) were classified as stage 2, while only one patient was classified as stage 3 (Figure 14).

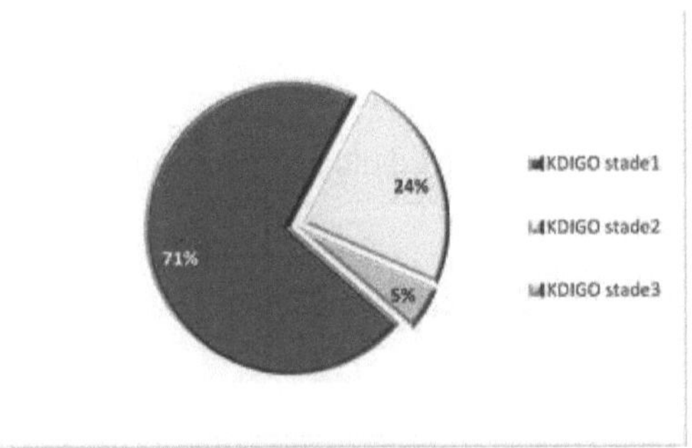

Figure 15: KDIGO classification of acute renal failure

1.10.2Consequences of acute renal failure

1.10.2.1 acute lung disease.

Of the twenty-one patients who developed CINP, five developed acute lung failure concomitant with a diuretic break, with four patients progressing well on diuretics.

1.10.2.2 Hyperkalemia

No patient had hyperkalaemia defined as a value of 5 mmol/l or more, regardless of the severity of ARL.

1.10.2.3 Use of hemodialysis

Recourse to hemodialysis was reported in a single diabetic patient with stage 4 CKD. Acute lung redema and anuria were the indications for urgent hemodialysis in this patient.

1.10.3Progression of acute renal failure

1.10.3.1 Recovery of renal function

Complete recovery of renal function was noted in 9 patients (42.8%) with a median time to return to normal creatinemia values of 5 days [2-10].

Five patients showed partial recovery, defined as a 25-50% fall in creatinemia during the follow-up period.

Only one patient, with stage 4 CKD, progressed to end-stage CKD and was transferred to the nephrology department for further management.

The outcome was unknown in the other patients because of the short hospital stay.

1.10.3.2 Length of stay

The median length of stay in the cardiology department in the event of the occurrence of

NPCI in our population was 5 days with an IQR of 25%-75% [3-10].

1.10.3.3 In-hospital deaths

The deaths of two patients were observed among those who developed NPCI, corresponding to 10% of this sample.

Both cases, free of CKD, presented with per-procedural hypotension associated with cardiogenic shock.

2 ANALYTICAL STUDY

2.1 Univariate analysis of factors associated with iodine contrast nephropathy

2.1.1 Epidemiological data

In our series, among the epidemiological data, only age >70 years was correlated with the occurrence of ARF associated with PCI, with a risk 3.2 times higher (p=0.032) than in other age groups, with a 95% CI [1.16 - 8.87] (Table XV).

TableXVI: Correlation between epidemiological data and the occurrence of NPCI

	NPCI		P
	0 UI	N ON	
Age (median)	65 years old	62 years old	0,091
Age > 70	8 (38%)	18(16%)	**0,032***
Age [50-69] years	12(57%)	79(70%)	0,226
Age <50	1(5%)	15(13%)	0,265
Men	14(67%)	79(70%)	0,723
Woman	7(33%)	33(29%)	

*Tac1енга55oc1ё a the occurrence of NPCI.   *NPCI: nёpКropa1Ьle assu^e lu contrast media юеез

2.1.2 Medical data

Among the antecedents observed in our study population, we found a statistical association between CKD and diabetic nephropathy with *the occurrence of* AKI associated with ICPs.

Indeed, *patients with CKD* had a 6.35-fold greater risk (95% CI [1.45 - 27.83], p=0.022) of developing AKI associated with ICPs compared with those with normal renal function.

Similarly, individuals with diabetic nephropathy had a 5-fold increased risk (95% CI [1.23 - 20.64], p=0.035) of developing CINP compared with those without this complication.

Among the medications administered simultaneously with the injection of PDC, the use of diuretics, particularly loop diuretics, and the administration of insulin were correlated with the occurrence of ARF associated with PCI. The risks of developing this complication were respectively 3 times higher for all diuretics (4 times higher for loop diuretics) and 2.73 times higher for insulin, compared with those not taking these drugs.

On the other hand, taking ARBs or betabiotics was associated with prevention of the risk of CINL, with a 3-fold greater probability of not developing this nephropathy.

The different correlations between anamnestic data and the occurrence of AKI associated with ICPs are shown in Table XVII.

Table XVIII: Correlation between anamnestic data and the occurrence of NPCI

	NPCI		P
	YES	NO	
Habits			
Active smoking	11(52%)	59(53%)	0,980
Background			
Diabetes	10(48%)	57(51%)	0,783
HTA	14(67%)	64(57%)	0,416
Dyslipidemia	9(43%)	36(32%)	0,341
Chronic renal failure	4(19%)	4(3,6%)	**0,022***
Diabetic nephropathy	4(19%)	5(4,5%)	**0,035***
Acute renal failure	2(9%)	4(4%)	0,240
PDC injection < 3 months	4(19%)	16(14%)	0,522
Number of cardiovascular risk factors > 2	19(90%)	95(85%)	0,737
Concomitant medication			
Diuretics	13(62%)	39(35%)	**0,02***
Spironolactone	3(14%)	14(12%)	0,737
Loop diuretics	9(43%)	18(16%)	**0,014***
Thiazide diuretics	4(19%)	17(15%)	0,744
BSRA	9(43%)	79(70%)	**0,014**
Diuretics and ASRB	6(29%)	34(30%)	0,870
Beta-agonists	12(57%)	89(79%)	**0,028**
Statins	19(90%)	104(93%)	0,658
PPI	19(90%)	90(80%)	0,364
ISGLT2	3(14%)	18(16%)	

Insulin	10(48%)	28(25%)	**0,035***
Metformin	4(19%)	17(15%)	0,744
Clopidogrel	19(90%)	98(87%)	1
Aspirin	16(76%)	101(90%)	0,134
NSAIDS	1(5%)	7(6%)	1

NSAIDs: non-steroidal anti-inflammatory drugs, RABS: renin angiotensin system blockers, PPIs: proton pump inhibitors, ISGLT2: SGLT2 pump inhibitors, NPCI: nёpKropaГble induced by contrast media, PDC: contrast media

***Factor associated with the development of CINP**   *CINP: nephropathy associated with iodine contrast products

2.1.3 Clinical data

Among the clinical data from the pre-procedural physical examination, dehydration was correlated with the occurrence of AKI associated with ICP, with a 13-fold higher risk of developing this nephropathy compared with normohydrate patients (IC95% [2.2-76.17]).

Similarly, patients with excess carbohydrates had a 4-fold greater risk of developing CINP compared with patients with normal carbohydrates (Table XIX).

TableXX: Correlation between clinical data and the occurrence of NPCI

	NPCI		P
	YES	NO	
Dehydration n(%)	4(19%)	2(2%)	0,006*
Overload n(%)	9(42,9%)	18(16,1%)	0,014*
PAS pre PCI (Median in mmHg)	130	130	0,897
PAD pre PCI (Median in mmHg)	75	75	0,997

***factor a55oc1ё to the occurrence of NPCI.**   *NPCI: nёpKropa1ble aззобёe to contrast media ^ёз

2.1.4 Biological data

Of the biological data requested in our study, only kalemia was not correlated with the occurrence of AKI associated with ICP (Table XXI).

Anemia and altered pre-procedural renal function were statistically associated with the occurrence of AKI in PCI patients with a 3.64-fold and 4-fold increased risk of developing CINP respectively (95% CI [1.39- 9.52], p=0.006), (95% CI [1.44-10.65], p=0.014).

We also found a statistically significant association between the neutrophil/lymphocyte ratio and the occurrence of AKI associated with ICP with an ROC threshold value >3.49 and a p<0.001.

Table XXII: Correlations between biological data and the occurrence of NPCI

NPCI			
	YES	NO	P
	Mediane		
Glomerular filtration rate pre-procedural	65,61 +/- 26	82,7 +/- 22	0,002*
Creatinine (umol/l)	90	78	0,013*
Altered renal function (n (%))	9(43%)	18(16%)	0,014*
Uree(mmol/l)	8,5	6	0,000*
Natremia(mmol/l)	136	138	0,002*
Kaliemie(mmol/l)	4,2	4,4	0,706
Hematocrit (%)	38%	41%	0,009*
Neutrophils(N) (/mm $)^3$	5795	5160	0,029*
Lymphocytes(L) (/mm $)^3$	1035	1810	0,001*
Neutrophil/lymphocyte ratio	4,8	2,7	0,000*
	Average +/-	Standard deviation	P
Hemoglobin (g/dl)	12 +/- 2,2	13,4 +/-1,83	0,017*
Anemia (n (%))	12(57%)	30(27%)	0,006*

*factor a55oc1ë a the occurrence of NPCI.   *NPCI: nëpKropa1ble a55oc1ëe to contrast media ^ë

2.1.5 Cardiographic echo data

According to the cardiographic echo data from our study, LVEF <40% was statistically associated with the occurrence of CINP with a 3.92-fold increased risk of developing it compared to patients with LVEF >40% (95% CI [1.44-10.65]) (TableXII).

It has been noted that patients with a dilated superior vena cava have a 4-fold increased risk of developing CINV compared with the rest of the patients (95% CI [1.18-14]).

Table XXIII: Correlations between echo-cardiographic data and the occurrence of NPCI

	NPCI	P

	YES	NO	
Mediane			
LVEF	**40%**	**57%**	**0,002***
	Number n(%)		
LVEF <40	**9(43%)**	**18(16%)**	**0,014***
LVEF 40%-49	6(29%)	13(12%)	0,08
LVEF > 50%	6(29%)	81(72%)	**0,000**
vcidilatde	5 (23,8%)	8 (7%)	
Non-dilated ICV	16 (76,2%)	104 (93%)	**0,033***

*LVEF: Left Ventricular Ejection Fraction, *NPCI: National Pacemaker Index

Nephropathy induced by ▪ contrast media

***Factor associated with the development of NPCI** *IVC: inferior vena cava

2.1.6 Procedural data

Table XXIV below shows that, in our study, the nature of the examination carried out, the approach used, HD instability during the procedure and the characteristics of the ICP used were statistically associated with the occurrence of ARF associated with ICPs.

Patients who underwent coronary angiography with primary angioplasty were 3.44 times more likely to develop ARF associated with PCI compared with the rest of the patients (95% CI [1.24-9.54]).

In terms of ICP characteristics, patients using iodixanol were 8.55 times more likely to develop ICP-associated ARF compared with patients using iohexol (95% CI [1.56-41.58]). In addition, ICP dose, the ratio of injected volume (ml)/clearance and iodine dose (g)/clearance were correlated with the occurrence of CINP with respective thresholds greater than 32.5 g (p = 0.04), 2.48 (p = 0.001), 0.74 (p = 0.001).

Furthermore, patients with a Mehran score >11 were 8.44 times more likely to develop AKI associated with PCI compared with those with a score <11 (95% CI [2.05 -34.76]).

Table XXV: Correlation between procedural data and occurrence of NPCI

NPCI	
Yes No	

			Number n(%)		P
Indicationof coronary angiography		Urgent indication <24h	14(67%)	76(68%)	
		Indication >24h	7(33%)	36(32%)	0,915
Examination	Nature of the act	Coronary angiography Only	4(19%)	49(44%)	**0,034**
		Coronary angiography and primary angioplasty	8(38%)	17(15%)	**0,028***
		Coronary angiography and ad hoc angioplasty	5(24%)	32(29%)	0,655
		Angioplasty	4(19%)	14(12%)	0,485
	Approach	Female	18(86%)	111(99%)	0,012
		Radial	3(14%)	3(2,7%)	**0,04**
	Clinical data	(HD instability)	3(14%)	1(1%)	**0,012***
Delaientre admission and act	Mediane		1 day	2 days	0,06
Contrast medium	Nature	Visipaque (Iodixanol…)	4(19%)	3(3%)	**0,012***
		Omnipaque	17(81%)	109(97%)	
	Volume	Mediane	120 ml	120 ml	0,052
	Dose	Mediane	36 g	30g	**0,04***
	Volume to brightness ratio	Mediane	2,48	1,25	**0,001***
	Dose/clearance ratio	Mediane	0,75	0,37	**0,001***
Result of coronary angiography		normal or infiltree	1(5%)	21(19%)	0,197
		Single-vessel disease	5(24%)	31(28%)	0,714
		Two-vessel disease	8(38%)	35(31%)	0,538
		Tritronvascular disease	7(33%)	25(22%)	0,279
Mehran score		Score > 11	5(23,8%)	4(3,6%)	**0,005***

*Factor associated with the development of NPCI   *BNPD: nephropathy associated with iodine contrast media

2.1.7 Evolving data

In our study, a correlation was found between length of hospital stay, in-hospital death and the occurrence of NPCI (table XXVI).

The presence of NPCI is associated with an increase in these parameters.

TableXXVII: Correlation between evolutionary data after the occurrence of NPCI

NPCI		P

	Yes	No	
Length of stay: median, IQR [25%-75%].	5 [3-10]	2[2-2]	**0,000***
Deaths inpatient n(%)	2 (10%)	0	**0,001***

*factor associated with the development of CINP *CINP: iodine contrast media-associated nephropathy

2.2 Multivariate analysis of factors associated with the occurrence of iodine contrast nephropathy

In the univariate analysis, several factors were identified as being predictive of the occurrence of AKI associated with ICP. To determine the independent factors for the occurrence of AKI, we chose to include in a multivariate analysis using binary logistic regression, the 30 factors of interest to the population as a whole. We found that chronic renal failure, a low left ventricular ejection fraction (<40%), dehydration, overload, primary angioplasty, high urea levels, a neutrophil/lymphocyte ratio >3.49, the use of iodixanol as a contrast agent and a dose/clash ratio >0.74 were independently associated with the occurrence of ARF associated with PCI.

In contrast, only LVEF >50% was identified as being independently associated with prevention of AKI associated with PCI. (Table XXVIII)

TableXXIX: Multivariate analysis of factors associated with the occurrence of NPCI

Factors associated with the occurrence of NPCI	P	Odds ratio	Intervalde 95% confidence	
			Lower	Superior
Anamnestic data				
AGE>70	0,159	2,832	0,665	12,065
Chronic rëna1e insufficiency	0,028*	5,544	1,202	25,558
Diuretics	0,403	1,738	0,476	6,344
Loop diuretics	0,262	2,090	0,577	7,572
Insulin	0,182	2,042	0,716	5,581
Clinical data				
OёзKy^a1a1юп	0,036*	8,442	1,155	61,723
Overload	0,037*	3,637	1,08	12,245
Instability HD	0,07	17,067	0,797	365,587
Ultrasound data				
LVEF < 40%.	0,008*	4,559	1,481	14,038

	P	Odds ratio	Intervalde 95% confidence	
Nature of the act				
Procë^re Coronary angiography + Primary angioplasty	0,019*	3,950	1,248	12,499
Biology				
Uree	0,022*	**1,423**	1,053	1,924
Creatinine	0,359	0,983	0,949	1,019
DFG prë procë^ra1e	0,568	1,013	0,970	1,057
Renal function aкёrёe	0,732	0,683	0,07	6,032
Natremie	0,125	1,197	0,951	1,506
Nǝmoglobin	0,313	1,170	0,862	1,588
Aпёт1e	0,126	2,475	0,776	7,894
Nǝmatocrit	0,220	1,434	0,806	2,550
Neutrophils	0,018*	**1,000**	0,900	1,000
Lymphocytes	0,125	1,001	1,000	1,002
Report neutrophils/lymphocytes >3,49	0,004*	**6,092**	1,784	20,797
PCI features				
Radial route	0,371	2,570	0,326	20,291
Iodinaxol(visipaque 320)	0,019*	**9,299**	1,438	60,153
PCI dose >32.5g	0,063	2,837	0,946	8,501
V/CL >2.48	0,103	4,090	0,754	22,188
D/CL >0.74	0,040*	**3,930**	1,004	15,383
Mehran score > 11	0,12	4	1	22,95

Factors associated with the prevention of a NPCI	P	Odds ratio	Intervalde 95% confidence	
			Lower	Superior
LVEF >50	0,002	11	2,403	50,314
Medicines				
BSRAA	0,299	2,018	0,536	7,601
Bëlabloянаn15	0,758	1,263	0,286	5,580

BSRA: Bloqueurs du systeme renine angiotensine neutrophiles/lymphocytes , PCI: produit de contraste iode clairance, VCI: veine cave inferrieure

DFG: Debit of 1 , V: volume injected

Glomerular filtration rate , N/L: Ratio , Dose: dose of contrast medium, CL :

*factor ^ëpe^aп! for the occurrence of NPCI.   *   NPCI: пёpKropa1ble asso^e to contrast media ^ë

Chapter 4

Advances in interventional cardiology have improved clinical diagnosis and patient management in recent years. However, most of these techniques are still dependent on the intravascular injection of iodine contrast medium, which has well-known toxicities, notably iodine contrast medium nephropathy. This condition, which has been recognised for some fifty years, is one of the main causes of acute renal failure in hospitals. It is thus associated with high hospital morbidity and mortality in both the short and long term.

Risk factors for iodine contrast nephropathy include both patient and procedure-related factors:

Patient-related factors: advanced age, diabetes, chronic or pre-existing renal failure, altered contractile function of the left ventricle, presence of anaemia, hypovolemia, use of nephrotoxic treatments.

Factors related to the procedure: (use of hyperosmolar contrast products, (use of excessive doses of iodinated contrast products, (repeated administration at short intervals, intra-arterial administration route and (urgent indication for the procedure.

Various scores have been developed to stratify the risk of this complication, in particular the Mehran clinical score.

This stratification has made it possible to optimise the management of patients at risk. Prevention remains the most effective means of managing iodine contrast nephropathy. Prevention depends essentially on the level of risk.

In this context, volume expansion is the only proven treatment for the prevention of iodine contrast nephropathy.

From a series of 133 patients explored by coronary angiography or treated by coronary angioplasty in the cardiology department of the Mongi Slim Hospital between April and June 2023, we propose to :

❖ Determining the incidence of ARF associated with iodine contrast products

❖ Identify predictive factors for the occurrence of contrast nephropathy in cardiology.

The inclusion criteria were all patients over 18 years of age who had undergone coronary angiography and/or coronary angioplasty at the cardiology department of the Mongi Slim Hospital during the study period. Non-inclusion criteria were patients with obstructive renal failure and chronic dialysis patients. Patients with missing data in the file were excluded, in particular pre- and post-procedural creatinine values.

The prevention protocol applied in this observational study is that adopted in the cardiology department, which mainly consists of rehydration with 9g/L NaCL, starting 24 hours before injection of the iodine contrast medium and continuing on the day of the procedure and 48 hours afterwards, while respecting the hydration status of the patients.

The median age of our patients was 63 years (28 to 82 years), with a predominance of males (70%). Subjects aged 70 or over represented 19% of patients.

The main cardiovascular risk factors were: smoking (53%), diabetes (50%), arterial hypertension (59%) and dyslipidemia (34%).

Twenty patients (15%) had undergone investigations requiring an injection of contrast products in the 3 months prior to coronary exploration.

Six patients (4.5%) showed signs of dehydration prior to contrast injection.

Eight patients (6%) had chronic renal failure.

Twenty-seven patients (20.3%) had left ventricular dysfunction.

The median pre-procedural creatinemia was 81pmol/l, with extremes ranging from 49 to 269pmol/l.

Anemia was present in 32% of patients.

The median Mehran risk score was 4, with extremes ranging from 0 to 21.

The interventional cardiology procedure consisted of coronary angiography in 41% of cases, primary angioplasty in 27% of cases, coronary angiography with ad-hoc angioplasty in 14% of patients and coronary angioplasty (elective) in 19% of cases.

The median volume of contrast medium injected was 100 ml, with extremes ranging from 30 to 500 ml.

The median volume/clearance ratio was 1.3, with extremes ranging from 0.4 to 15.6, while the median iodine dose in grams/clearance ratio was 0.4, with extremes ranging from 0.12 to 5.

The overall incidence of contrast nephropathy was 16%, or 21 patients.

In a multivariate study, the occurrence of this complication was significantly associated with the following risk factors:

❖ Chronic renal failure (p=0.028 odds ratio: 5.544 95% CI [1.202-25.558])

❖ Hydration status (dehydration: p=0.036 odds ratio: 8.442 IC 95% [1.155-61.723] and overload: p=0.037 odds ratio: 3.637 IC 95% [1.0812.245])

❖ Left ventricular ejection fraction less than 40% (p=0.008 odds ratio: 4.559 IC 95% [1.481-14.038])

❖ Primary angioplasty (p=0.019 odds ratio: 3.950 IC 95% [1.24812.499])

❖ Urea (p=0.022 odds ratio: 1.423 95% CI [1.053-1.924])

❖ Neutrophil/lymphocyte ratio >3.49 (p=0.004 odds ratio: 6.092 IC95% [1.784-20.797])

❖ Dose/clearance ratio >0.74 (p=0.040 odds ratio: 3.930 IC 95% [1.004-15.383])

In contrast, only a left ventricular ejection fraction >50% was found to be independently associated with prevention of acute renal failure associated with iodine contrast media (p=0.002 odds ratio: 11IC 95% [2.403-50.314].

The limitations of our study were as follows:

❖ The retrospective and mono-centric nature of the study

❖ The short observation period

❖ The number of patients included was not as large.

❖ Serum creatinine was only measured pre-procedure and at D2-3. Late-onset NPCI was possible up to D10 and was under-diagnosed.

❖ Serum creatinine is a non-specific marker for assessing the effectiveness of preventive measures against CINP.

At the end of our study, we suggest :

❖ Identify the risk factors for the development of contrast nephropathy related to the patient and the procedure,

❖ Prefer iso or hypo-osmolar iodine contrast media

❖ Use the smallest possible volume of contrast

❖ Incorporate a more objective measure of contrast medium volume, such as maximum allowable contrast volume or the ratio of contrast medium volume to creatinine clearance.

❖ Continue to take renin-angiotensin system blockers before injecting contrast media, particularly in coronary patients, for their beneficial effects on cardiac remodelling.

REFERENCES

1. Houssaini TS. Prevention de la toxicite des produits de contraste iodes en cardiologie interventionnelle Prevention of contrast induced nephropathy in interventional cardiology. 2010;

2. Azzalini L, Spagnoli V, Ly HQ. Contrast-Induced Nephropathy: From Pathophysiology to Preventive Strategies. Canadian Journal of Cardiology. 1 Feb 2016;32(2):247-55.

3. Ronco F, Tarantini G, McCullough PA. Contrast induced acute kidney injury in interventional cardiology: an update and key guidance for clinicians. RCM. 30 March 2020;21(l):9-23.

4. Humbert A, Kissling S, Teta D. Contrast medium nephropathy. Rev Med Suisse. 5 June 2013;389(22):1222-8.

5. Tsai TT, Patel UD, Chang Tl, Kennedy KF, Masoudi FA, Matheny ME, et al. Contemporary Incidence, Predictors, and Outcomes of Acute Kidney Injury in Patients Undergoing Percutaneous Coronary Interventions. JACC Cardiovasc Interv. Jan 2014;7(l):l-9.

6. De Laforcade L, Bobot M, Bellin MF, Clement O, Grange S, Grenier N, et al. ESUR recommendations on the use of contrast media: practice survey, review and commentary by the CJN, FIRN and SFNDT. Nephrologie & Therapeutique. Apr 2021;17(2):80-91.

7. Notice. Kidney International Supplements, March 2012;2(l):l.

8. Ad-hoc working group of ERBP, Fliser D, Laville M, Covic A, Fouque D, Vanholder R, et al. A European Renal Best Practice (ERBP) position statement on the Kidney Disease Improving Global Outcomes (KDIGO) clinical practice guidelines on acute kidney injury: part 1: definitions, conservative management and contrast-induced nephropathy. Nephrol Dial Transplant, Dec 2012;27(12):4263-72.

9. Mghaieth F, Ayari J, Ben Rejeb R, Mbarki S, Farhati A, Larbi N, et al [Contrast-induced nephropathy after cardiac catheterization: a prospective study of 180 patients], Tunis Med. Apr 2012;90(4):320-7.

10. Laroussi L, Halima AB, Houmed A, Bennour E, Haj ZE, Boukhris M, et al. Iodixanol versus Iopromide in patients at high riskfor contrast induced nephropathy: IO2 contrast study Iodixanol versus Iopromide in patients at high risk of contrast-induced nephropathy: IO2 contrast study. 2018;

11. Spagnoli V, Azzalini L, Tadros VX, Picard F, Ly HQ. Contrast-induced nephropathy: an update. Annals of Cardiology and Angeiology. Apr 2016;65(2):87-94.

12. Summary of product characteristics - OMNIPAQUE 300 mg d'I/mL, solution injectable - Base de données publique des medicaments [Internet], [cite 22 mai 2024]. Available from: https://base-donnees-publique.medicaments.gouv.fr/affichageDoc.php?specid=65106581&typedoc=R

13. Summary of product characteristics - VISIPAQUE 320 mg d'I/mL, solution injectable - Base de données publique des medicaments [Internet], [cite 22 mai 2024]. Available from: https://base-donnees-publique.medicaments.gouv.fr/affichageDoc.php?specid=60567418&typedoc=R

14. Livio F, Biollaz J, Burnier M. Estimation de la fonction renale par l'equation MDRD : interet et limites pour l'adaptation des doses de medicaments. Rev Med Suisse. 26 Nov 2008;181(43):2596-600.

15. Mehran R, Aymong ED, Nikolsky E, Lasic Z, Iakovou I, Fahy M, et al. A simple risk score for prediction of contrast-induced nephropathy after percutaneous coronary intervention: Development and initial validation. Journal of the American College of Cardiology. 6 Oct 2004;44(7):1393-9.

16. Gariani K, Tran C. Glycaemoglobin: a new screening tool? Rev Med Suisse. 8 June 2011;298(22):1238-42.

17. WHO_NMH_NHD_MNM_ll.l_eng.pdf [Internet], [cited 22 May 2024]. Available from:

https://iris.who.int/bitstream/handle/10665/85839/WHO_NMH_NHD_MNM_II.I_eng.pdf

18.   MAR_D1_RBPM Hypertention arterielle de l'adulte.pdf [Internet], [cite 22 May 2024]. Available on   :
https://extranet.who.int/ncdccs/Data/MAR_Dl_RBPM%20Hypertention%20arteri%C3%A9lle%
20of%20adult.pdf

19.   Classification des insuffisances cardiaques et demarche etiologique [Internet], [cite 22 May 2024].
Available from: https://www.larevuedupraticien.fr/article/classification-des-   heart-failure-and-etiological-
approach

20.   I Extracellular dehydration (ECD) - [Renal physiology and physiopathology] [Internet], [cite 22 May 2024].
Available from: https://cuen.fr/lmd/spip.php2rubrique96

21.   III Intracellular dehydration (ICD) - [Renal physiology and physiopathology] [Internet], [cite 22 May 2024].
Available from: https://cuen.fr/lmd/spip.php2rubrique98

22.   Serveaux M, Burnier M, Kissling S. Interpretation of volemia in acute renal failure. Rev Med Suisse. 26 Feb
2014;419:474-9.

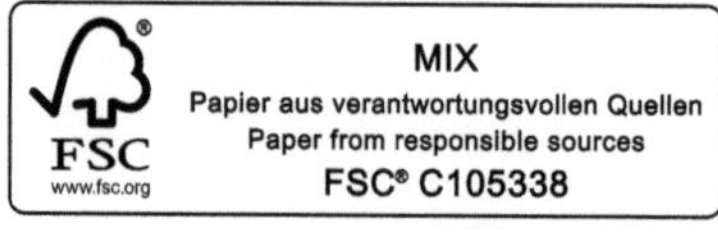

Printed by Books on Demand GmbH, Norderstedt / Germany